WEIGHT WATCHERS
101 More SECRETS FOR SUCCESS

Macmillan · USA

MACMILLAN
A Simon & Schuster Macmillan Company
1633 Broadway
New York, NY 10019-6785

Copyright © 1996 by Weight Watchers International, Inc.
All rights reserved. No part of this book may be reproduced or transmitted in any form
by any means, electronic or mechanical, including photocopying, recording, or by any
information storage and retrival system, without permission from the Publisher.
MACMILLAN is a registered trademark of Macmillan, Inc.
WEIGHT WATCHERS is a registered trademark of Weight Watchers International, Inc.

Library of Congress Cataloging-in-Publication Data
Weight Watchers 101 more secrets of success.
p. cm.
ISBN 0-02-861499-2
1. Weight loss.   2. Weight loss—Psychological aspects.
I. Weight Watchers International
RM222.2.W2986 1997
613.2'5—dc20   96-24780
                                CIP

Interior design by Anne Scatto and Andrea Weinreb

Introduction

If you've ever tried to lose weight, you know how important it is to have support—someone in your corner who cheers you on, offers a helping hand and always has a great tip or a word of encouragement that's tailor-made for the situation.

At Weight Watchers, the weekly meetings provide a supportive environment for members to share the problems they have encountered, as well as the solutions they discovered. Sometimes, though, you need support *now,* and that's why we've created *Weight Watchers 101 More Secrets for Success.* Carry this little volume in your purse, pocket, briefcase or backpack. When you need a brilliant idea or just a simple boost, flip through its pages. You're sure to find just the right words.

Work on improving your self-image. Simple things like keeping your shoes shined, your nails polished and your clothes neatly pressed will reward you with a good feeling every time you pass a mirror or see your reflection in a store window.

Rethink the way you measure success. In addition to weight loss, have you learned new and better eating habits? Do you feel healthier? Can you wear a smaller size? Can you handle stressful situations without food? All these things contribute to success.

Low-fat foods can be a mixed blessing! The absence of fat is often compensated for by extra sugar, so the total calories are not always lower. Make a point of reading labels to be sure that you are getting the best nutritional "buy."

Hot-air popped popcorn is a real food bonus: 3 full cups provide 2 grams of fiber and absolutely no fat! While the popcorn is still warm, season it with butter-flavored sprinkles and onion or garlic powder for a crunchy, savory snack.

Speak up for yourself! In restaurants, be pleasant but clear in requesting what you want: dressing on the side, food broiled, no butter, steamed vegetables, and so on. If you are served something you don't want, feel free to ask for a substitute. You'll find that most restaurants are accustomed to these requests and happy to honor them.

Going on a trip? Make a "survival kit" containing individual packets of nonfat salad dressing, sugar substitutes, broth mixes, sugar-free hot cocoa mix and mini-boxes of raisins.

𝒫ack pre-measured servings of ready-to-eat cereal, pretzels, graham crackers and dried fruits in resealable plastic bags for your office desk drawer.

𝓑lanch raw vegetables to bring out their most brilliant colors. Then make a healthful dip by stirring hot salsa or whole-grain mustard into plain nonfat yogurt.

Squeeze fresh lemon juice on a baked white potato, or sprinkle cinnamon and ground nutmeg on a baked sweet potato. If your office has a microwave, these potatoes can make quick, nonfat, high-fiber lunches.

*E*nhance a frozen low-calorie entrée by adding more vegetables or serving it on a bed of steamed greens.

Walk to the newsstand for your morning paper instead of having it delivered. If your shopping list is short, hook a basket over your handlebars and bike to the store.

If you're not accustomed to regular activity, start out slowly, even if it's just a walk around the block.
Gradually increase the time and intensity. If you're pressed for time and can't do a full 30-minute workout, try to fit in three 10-minute workouts over the course of the day.

Do your grocery shopping after *a meal or snack—shopping when you're hungry is an invitation to pick up the wrong foods.*

*A*lways set a place for yourself and eat at the table, not in front of the open refrigerator, over the sink, or while you're clearing up after a meal.

*T*uck a bottle of water in your purse or tote bag so it's always handy. Aim to drink 8 glasses each day; once you get into the habit, you won't even have to think about it.

Write down everything you eat, even if it's just a small amount. You will be amazed at what you might be "forgetting" to count.

Discover spaghetti squash; when cooked, it turns into strands. Use it to stretch pasta portions; it also tastes delicious on its own, topped with tomato sauce.

Top breakfast toast with unsweetened applesauce and a sprinkle of cinnamon, or spread with nonfat cream cheese and mashed banana for a fruity morning treat.

Although some people are successful in losing weight on their own, many find that a support group helps a lot. Being around others who can provide advice and encouragement often helps you to get through a rough spot. It also feels wonderful to share your successes!

Don't be a breakfast-skipper. It truly is the most important meal of the day and helps you avoid a dangerous mid-morning slump just as the coffee and doughnut cart is coming down the hall.

Are you eating the right foods in the wrong portions?
An easy route to weight loss is learning to "eyeball" appropriate
size portions; for instance, 3 ounces of meat is about
the size of a deck of cards; 1 ounce of hard cheese is
the size of your thumb.

If you're still cooking with salt, begin to reduce it gradually until you become accustomed to the real flavors of food. Use lemon or lime juice, flavored vinegars, or herbs and spices to perk up your meals.

*A*re you eating the right foods in the wrong portions? An easy route to weight loss is learning to "eyeball" appropriate size portions; for instance, 3 ounces of meat is about the size of a deck of cards; 1 ounce of hard cheese is the size of your thumb.

If you're still cooking with salt, begin to reduce it gradually until you become accustomed to the real flavors of food. Use lemon or lime juice, flavored vinegars, or herbs and spices to perk up your meals.

*I*nstead of sauteing onions, garlic, celery and carrots in oil, save calories by sprinkling them with water and softening for a minute in the microwave before adding them to a recipe.

*C*ook with nonstick cookware, lightly sprayed with nonstick cooking spray. Preheat pans briefly before adding food to them.

Take advantage of the seasons to enjoy a variety of exercise. In the summer: swim, bicycle, canoe, play softball or volleyball or try hiking. In the winter, go ice-skating, sledding, or cross-country skiing. On stormy stay-at-home days, work out to a favorite exercise video or put on your favorite music and dance.

Indulge a little! Having an occasional small helping of a favorite food will keep you from feeling deprived. If sweets are your thing, for just 50 calories you can enjoy two chocolate kisses, five jelly beans, or ten chocolate-covered peanuts.

*I*nstead of serving yourself from the platter or bowl, portion your food directly onto your plate from the stove. When you have finished your meal or snack, wrap leftovers and store them out of sight!

Feeling stressed? A good workout can do a lot to relieve tension and stretch aching muscles. Contrary to old wives' tales, exercise doesn't make you hungry or tired but actually revs up your energy level.

*E*at a wide variety of foods to avoid boredom. Try a new fruit or vegetable at least once a week.

*G*ot an urge to splurge? Wait 20 minutes before you indulge; it might just go away.

Buying lunch at the deli? Order your sandwich on whole-grain bread for more fiber and ask for just 2 ounces of meat. Skip the butter and mayo; instead ask for mustard and a juicy pickled sweet red pepper.

*H*aving dinner out? Make friends with your waitperson and ask to have half your meal put into a doggie bag before it's even served to you.

When eating out, explore the appetizer section of your menu. One or two "starters" and a salad gives you a chance to taste more things and keep the portions under control.

On your next restaurant trip with a friend, ask if you can share a lunch or dinner entrée. Even if there is a small surcharge, it will still be cheaper than two meals, both in cost and calories!

*I*f your supermarket doesn't stock the ingredients you need, ask the manager to order them. Most grocers will be happy to have your suggestions as it means they will be serving their customers better.

Never give up! A momentary indiscretion does not a failure make. Forge ahead with renewed vigor and commitment.

For recipes calling for eggs, look for nonfat egg substitute in the refrigerator or freezer case. Unless you need just the whites or a hard-cooked egg, you'll save lots of fat without sacrificing taste.

$\mathcal{M}$ake sure that your travel plans include a call to your airline at least 24 hours before your flight. You can order a special meal that meets your needs at absolutely no extra cost.

*S*hare the nutritional knowledge you've gained with friends and family—eating better is generally a universal goal.

*I*nvolve your family in your activity plans. Make today the time to take a bicycle ride, a walk in the park, play a game of touch football or row across the lake. Exercise doesn't just have to be workouts at the gym.

Make success a self-fulfilling prophecy. Start out with an "I can do this" attitude and reward yourself for each small victory. Keeping a journal is a good way to chart your progress. When you reread the pages, you'll be surprised at how far you've come.

*I*f you're going on a car trip, invest in a cooler and stock it with snacks that fit into your food plan. The fewer stops you make at fast food spots along the highway, the better.

𝓡ediscover your kitchen! Plan to try one new recipe each week and get points for being a low-cal, low-fat chef.

Who ever said that breakfast had to be juice, cereal and milk? If you're hungry in the morning, it's perfectly okay to have a bowl of soup, a sandwich or some pasta. Just rearrange the rest of your day to balance out your meal plan.

Reward yourself for achieving even small goals, but take care to make them nonfood treats. A CD you've wanted, a massage, a new blouse or a ticket to a special concert will make you feel pampered and special. You deserve it!

While you're working on weight loss, set some other goals that are easily measurable and attainable: taking a longer walk, writing a letter to an old friend, volunteering at a hospital or shelter, helping someone learn English as a second language. It's a great feeling to give of yourself.

*G*o green. There is increasing evidence that even an occasional vegetarian diet is healthful. Plan to have a non-meat dinner once or twice a week. Discover what you can do with tofu, grains and beans; you'll be pleasantly surprised.

Take advantage of precut vegetables in the produce department; new packaging technology creates a favorable climate for vegetables so that freshness, vitamins and minerals are retained.

For a fast and flavorful Mexican fish sauce: Bring 1 cup salsa and ¼ cup chopped cilantro to a boil; spoon over broiled or grilled fish fillets and sprinkle with Monterey Jack cheese.

*F*eed other hungers: Go to a museum and feast your eyes on art; treat your ears to a live concert or a CD. Satisfy a hearty appetite for knowledge with a class or workshop.

Don't postpone buying attractive clothing,
getting a great haircut or other nice-to-do things.
You deserve to look and feel good
every day of your life.

𝓑elieve in yourself. Don't beat yourself up. Instead, examine your lapses for the lessons they can teach you: Did I let myself get too hungry? Stressed? Tired? What can I do differently?

Walk for an hour. Don't worry about how far you're going or how fast. Stop whenever you like to window shop or lean against a tree. One rule: No sitting allowed!

Are you watching TV or just sitting in front of the screen?
Become a television critic and choose what you want to see.
Use the free time you gain to exercise with a fitness tape.

*F*ocus on how to really relax. Carve out a bit of time in your day to do something you really enjoy, or just do nothing at all.

*S*ilence the inner brat. Acknowledge the voice that demands you buy the doughnut; tell her that you might do that one day but right now you're having whole-wheat toast.

𝒜 "why me" attitude can get in the way of progress. Avoid self-pity, recognize that you are not alone and acknowledge all the help you are receiving.

*E*nlist your family in your efforts. Explain your food plan to them. That way they'll understand that when the kids want ice cream, your husband craves chips and everyone wants a fast-food dinner, you won't be joining them.

*E*xperiment in the kitchen. Create lighter versions of family favorites; chances are they'll never detect the low-fat cheese in their casserole or the low-fat mayonnaise in the potato salad.

*M*ake everyone over the age of 12 in your household responsible for their own "treats." Once you stop buying the candy and the chips, they may not continue to indulge themselves.

*D*ump the guilt. Can't iron a shirt because you have to go to exercise class? Won't make fried chicken because of the fat? This isn't selfish, it's necessary.

𝓕ind and buy a non-fattening food for all your cravings: pickles for salty, caramel-flavored rice cakes for sweet, yogurt for creamy and pretzels for crunchy.

*I*f a food is out of your control, don't buy it.
Unless you can eat just one cookie, pass up the box.

When you go to a party, arm yourself by bringing one course. Volunteer to bring a platter of vegetables with a low-fat dip, a big bowl of crisp green salad with a nonfat dressing, or a bountiful fresh fruit salad. Then watch everyone enjoy your contribution.

$\mathcal{A}$void potentially hazardous encounters. If you are invited to a make-your-own-sundae party, it might be wise to pass. Food-laden occasions tend to be booby-traps.

Become risk-averse. Find a shop for your morning coffee that does not also offer 37 varieties of doughnuts; don't keep a candy dish on your desk for visits from co-workers. Recognize temptation and cut it off at the pass.

𝒫lan a back-up option for your activity plan.
If it snows, your walking program may be cancelled.
Have a workout video or a jump rope ready so you don't
miss a day's exercise.

*S*atisfaction is deepest and most enduring when inspired by your own achievements. When you learn to balance pleasure with pride, satisfaction is total. Look for satisfaction in experiences, not from food.

$\mathcal{F}$ocus attention on the changes in your body, not the ups and downs of the scale. When you feel comfortable tucking in your blouse or wearing a belt, or when you can zip up a skirt you couldn't wear before, that's real progress.

*D*iscover the power of visualization. Create a "coach" to be at your side: imagine that you have her wonderful eating habits, such as knowing how to order in a restaurant or how to negotiate a fat-laden buffet.
Then "hear" her congratulate you on your choices.

*M*ake appropriate choices at a party and remember that no one is paying as much attention to your plate as you are.

*R*esist food pushers. A polite "No, thank you" should be sufficient but keep in mind that they, not you, are being thoughtless.

𝒥f your hostess really cares about you, she will not be offended if you decline her special cheesecake. Or, tell her that you are really full but would like to take it home for later. (Find someone to give it to or dispose of it before you get home.)

$\mathcal{B}$ecome a playwright and write yourself a script.
In your mind, imagine the social gathering you have been invited
to and how you will avoid unplannned eating.

Stress is a common overeating trigger. Don't eat to give yourself a break. Clear your head with a brisk walk, a tall glass of water or a call to a friend.

𝓜ake a mental "after" picture. What will you look like after you've lost weight? Visualize the changes after ten, twenty or thirty pounds. What will you be able to wear?

Be more flexible about mealtimes. If you've had a stressful day, take some time to relax: go for a walk, play with your dog or soak your feet before tackling dinner.

Spend mealtimes eating. Watching TV, opening the mail or paying bills distracts you from the taste and pleasure of your food. It's also hard to know when you're full if you're not paying attention.

*B*e more flexible about mealtimes. If you've had a stressful day, take some time to relax: go for a walk, play with your dog or soak your feet before tackling dinner.

Spend mealtimes eating. Watching TV, opening the mail or paying bills distracts you from the taste and pleasure of your food. It's also hard to know when you're full if you're not paying attention.

Weight loss, unlike other projects, takes ongoing effort. Exercise can help speed the process, and with each pound you lose, you get closer to your goal.

*E*nvision the big picture. There will be days when you go off your food plan and others when you really pour it on at the gym. Neither of these extremes will make or break your progress; what matters is how these days add up over the long haul.

*G*et rhythm. Get used to a regular exercise routine
and it will become as automatic as brushing your teeth.
Vary your activities to avoid boredom;
spirited dancing can be as aerobic as a step class.

*G*et enough rest. Even if this means you do not accomplish everything you planned for the day, make sure you get enough sleep. You will be unlikely to exercise or eat well if you are overtired.

When you are traveling, be prepared to wait. Bring a book, a personal stereo, knitting, or some other project to the airport or train station and avoid trips to the snack bar.

*A*way from home? Start your day in control by choosing fruit or cereal from the room service menu or breakfast buffet. That way, one-third of your day is already a success.

*S*hop the condiment aisle. Herbs, spices, relishes, flavored vinegars and mustards can add excitement to grilled, steamed, poached or broiled foods.

𝓑rowse in a low-calorie, low-fat cookbook for something you've never tasted before. It might be tofu, tempeh, orange roughy or cilantro. Try one ingredient in a new recipe every week.

*I*nvent a low-calorie, low-fat meal that incorporates your favorite tastes. Learn which flavorings typify the foods you like: coriander and curry for Indian; cilantro and chiles for Mexican; basil and oregano for Italian.

The only way you can fail at weight loss is by giving up.
If at first you don't succeed, ask what went wrong.
Once you know this, you are already one step closer to your goal.

Accept your failures, but don't become them.
If you missed going to the gym last week, you might have acted in
a lazy fashion but that does not mean that you are lazy.
And what's more, today is a whole new day.

Keep in mind that failure is hard to maintain.
Even a small success, such as refusing a second helping,
is enough to ruin a record of perfect failure.

*K*eep a diary of all your experiences, the good and the bad.
Then record what you've learned from them.
Remember the ones you want to repeat and the ones to avoid.

$\mathcal{B}$e a picky eater. Always ask yourself if this food is worth the calories, fat or sodium. If you find yourself unsure, take a pass.

*G*et more from less. Enjoy one small piece of deluxe chocolate instead of a whole third-rate candy bar.

Can you trace your extra pounds to those times when you ate even though you were not really hungry? Learn the difference between true hunger and "wanting to eat something."

What are you hungry for? The more specific the hunger, the more likely it is to be a craving.

Be on the lookout for "food triggers." Were you hungry before you passed the bakery with its seductive aromas? If not, you're being led by the nose.

*Don't allow the clock to decide your mealtime.
If you're not hungry for lunch at noon, then eat an hour later.*

*D*on't try to make up for bad days. A week of overeating followed by a week of starving will only make you feel deprived and set you up for a repeat of overindulging.
Just get back on track and pick up where you left off.

𝓑e responsible but don't be ashamed. Instead of blaming the heaping buffet table for your overload, or hating yourself for having no willpower, consider that *you* put yourself in a difficult situation. Ask yourself how you can do better the next time. Then act on it.

*S*hare. You're not the only person who ate her way to the bottom of the ice-cream carton and then cried all night. Confiding in someone who really listens will help.

Take a long view. Your weight gain didn't occur in a few weeks but probably over a period of time. Give yourself the opportunity to lose the weight just as gradually.
You can do it!